THE BODY TYPE DIET
Food Combining for a Leaner You!

Robert Adamo
Certified Nutritional Consultant

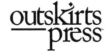
outskirts
press

Table of Contents

To my readers,

Imagine being in control of your eating habits; losing weight; becoming more fit and firm; having sustained energy; feeling your very best; and becoming healthier overall. Well, with this book, you'll stop imagining and start making these things your reality!

Welcome to **The Body Type Diet**, a unique nutritional system that is completely individualized for your specific body type. It is designed to teach you how to find the right food combinations for your body. This program will help you lose unwanted pounds and keep them off, achieve your fitness goals, reach an ideal target weight in the process, and acquire knowledge and understanding of a nutritional system that works for you.

This knowledge and understanding, combined with healthier eating patterns and exercise habits, will effortlessly—before you know it—become a part of your everyday routine.

And the results are fast. Each and every day you'll find yourself becoming leaner as your metabolism safely speeds up, you drop fat, and experience dramatic results that will change your life.

How do I know? Because of my education in things such as nutrition, sports medicine, and physiology, in addition to my twenty-five-plus years working one-on-one with thousands of individuals from all walks of life. I've worked with people of all ages, sizes, and shapes, folks who reached out in a hopeful effort not only to look better but also to feel better, just like you and me.

My motivation for writing this book was my own surprising sucess discovering what foods worked together to help me achieve my ideal weight. My motivation was simply this: I strongly believe this program will help you because I have a passion for what I do and have seen my nutrition advice and guidance work time and time again.

But before we begin, I'd like to congratulate you for taking the first step in improving your health and well-being. Starting right now, from the top of this page to the back cover of this book, you are my new client. Together, day by day, week after week, we will turn your dreams into a lean, healthy reality, celebrating the inevitable, dramatic changes that will take place with your body and in your life.

Consider me your body-type coach. I'm with you every step of the way.

Today I am happy to say that The Body Type Diet has changed my lifestyle of eating as well as that of my kids. The way we feed our kids is paramount to their healthy life. What is so nice about the Body Type Diet is that is family friendly. I cannot tell you the number of female clients who thank me for their husbands having lost weight and becoming healthier because of the great dinner combinations they have been eating.

What really makes this diet different from any other diet out there? I am not going to explain it in one paragraph. Let me just say other diets have a beginning and no end. This diet has a beginning and an end. The end result is you lose weight, feel great, and are in control. Look below at the two pictures of me at 200 pounds. The reason I am showing you these photos is that once I experienced the results of The Body Type Diet, my life changed for the better. Anyone who has a so-called diet program must walk the

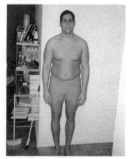

200 pounds 35 percent bodyfat

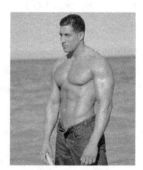

200 pounds 7 percent body fat

walk and not just talk the talk. I can talk science to you all day, but I can show you physically how that science changed my body. I am not going to lecture you in a lab coat and profess to have the next best thing, like many professionals do. I am going to passionately help you feel fit and healthy.

Now let's take a moment to congratulate you for coming this far. You see, the starting point of your journey is a desire to become healthy and fit, which you've already got! You've gone beyond the passive desire, and you've taken action. You've already taken steps to control your health and body—to overcome obstacles and make your future much brighter.

Meet Robert Adamo, Your Body Type Coach

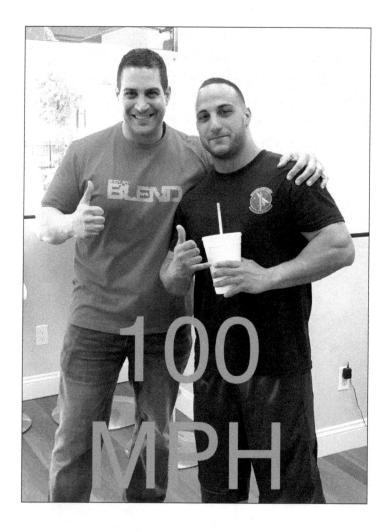

You have heard about *The South Beach Diet*, Weight Watchers, Atkins, *You on a Diet*, *The Keto Diet*, and the fasting diet, so who is Robert Adamo? I know you've never heard of Robert

Adamo, but consider me your buddy, and if you follow the suggestions in this book, you will thank Robert Adamo in the end.

Before we jump into The Body Type Diet, it's important for you to know me—to know that I have been where you are, and that I personally followed this plan and still do to this day. In my earlier years, I searched for various ways to lose weight and found that many books were useful in the promise of a new beginning. They told me what foods to eat and provided some good nutritional information, but none lived up to their billing. None provided me with the three things I needed most: 1) a motivating coach to guide me along the journey, 2) the secrets of how to eat for my specific body requirement, and 3) a nutrition program that becomes a lifestyle. For that reason, it gives me such great pleasure to be able to provide these things for you in this book.

The power of The Body Type Diet comes down to this: I know the body, I know food combining, and I know how to help people get the results they need. It was really the success of my nutrition program for twenty years that led to The Body Type Diet.

I became a certified nutritional consultant and supplement specialist and have devoted the past twenty-five years to studying nutrition and the body. It is my passion. I am currently a member of the American Association of Nutritional Consultants.

My experience with working with thousands of clients taught me that there is much more to nutrition than deprivation. There is a great deal of science involved in nutrition, and the lack of proper knowledge sets people up for failure.

When I was young, I ate a great deal of junk foods and fast foods. My parents fed us whatever there was to eat, and because of that, I was sick all the time and became overweight.

That path was destined to ignore the most basic of facts: what we eat has a biochemical effect on our body, and different foods have different biochemical effects. In fact some foods eaten in combination can have a biochemical effect on our bodies that helps us lose weight and achieve better health.

After four more years studying nutrition and successfully changing my body from a soft 260 pounds to a tight, lean 210 pounds, I took my nose out of the books, got my butt out of the library, and embarked on a journey to teach people everything I had learned. I wanted to share how I went about transforming my body and my life with those who were curious and seeking change.

I realized that simple things people were doing were working against them. For example, many were skipping breakfast. Those unfamiliar with nutrition—which includes most people—might not understand that ignoring that first meal of the day immediately shuts down your metabolism, and with your metabolism shut off, you cannot lose weight or burn fat.

People were eating carbs (also known as carbohydrates) alone, such as having just a bowl of oatmeal. Unfortunately, carbohydrates turn to sugar in the body and extra sugar turns to fat.

Working with clients I realized I was not only helping them understand why they had become overweight in the first place, but also quite honestly teaching them the right way to eat.

That is why I created The Body Type Diet.

Over the years, it's proven to be a tried and true, very simple program for losing weight quickly with long-term maintainable results. This book approaches the topic of nutrition and weight loss from an entirely different perspective than the typical low-calorie-diet approach. With my program you get to eat and eat a lot, dropping pounds in the process, and you'll learn that eating small, frequent meals in the right combinations is pivotal to your success.

Based on my years of experience with people of all shapes and sizes, I know if you follow the program outlined in this book for your body type, you will lose—in just twelve weeks—enough weight to boost your self-esteem and prove once and for all that you're finally on the right track.

You won't find calorie counting, food measuring, quick fixes or gimmicks in these pages, and I'm not going to insist you eat only grapefruit or vegetable juice or restrict yourself to 800 calories a day or completely eliminate carbohydrates.

What you will find are easy-to-follow basics about what you can do to get the results you want as well as customized menus to help you drop pounds instantly. And the only thing I'll insist you do is an exclusive, very easy Body Type Test.

Everyone is metabolically different. Some people can eat a bowl of pasta and not gain weight, while others like me eat pasta and gain five pounds. To succeed and enjoy long-term results, you must select the right meals for your body type. Doing so will allow you to lose weight quickly.

An understanding of your body type—gained from the results of the Body Type Test—is not only pivotal to the success of this program, but absolutely necessary for you to discover the right meals and quickly jump-start your own natural fat-burning weight-loss machine.

In following your customized food plan—meals comprised of great foods in great combinations—there is no room for error. You automatically and naturally consume the best nutrients in the right ratios.

You'll discover, as I did, that eating and exercising according to your body type will drop the weight and keep it off.

I'll also teach you about certain foods that actually improve your skin, helping you look and feel younger, and that a diet rich in fruits and nuts helps improve your immune system, while your digestive system benefits from a diet packed with vegetables.

As you and I work together you will learn how you can make The Body Type Diet a part of your everyday life. Once you have all this information—from the self-test, to discovering your body type, to specified meal combinations—you can stop the nutritional roller coaster that has been defining your life.

Every time I tried a diet and failed, I, like most people, felt like a failure, as if I somehow let myself down. I wasted time hoping that the next great diet would come along and give me the answer. Because of what I've discovered and made a part of my everyday life, though, I now feel better than I have in years. Now it's your turn.

In fact, it's time to get off of that diet roller coaster once and for all.

Chapter 1

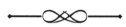

About the Body Type Diet

No two bodies are alike. There is no "one size fits all." Each of us responds differently to what we eat because of the way food chemically breaks down in our bodies. Just as your body undergoes changes, so should your food and exercise plan, but many weight loss programs refuse to recognize this fact. Most, in fact, appear to be based on the premise that "everyone is the same," resulting in a lot of short-term weight-loss successes, but very few long-term results.

The Body Type Diet was created with the understanding that everyone is physiologically and anatomically different with each person having a unique genetic makeup. The customized programs you'll find in these pages—designed specifically for each body type—not only achieve quick weight loss that lasts, but also help you maintain a lifestyle centered around healthy nutrition.

In truth, the formula for losing weight and keeping it off comes down to finding the right food combinations that help you ignite your natural fat-burning machine on a biochemical level. This process begins with discovering your body type.

Of course, some of you may want to immediately know *"What should I eat to lose weight?"* That's fine. Take the Body Type Diet Test—a necessary step in discovering your body type—and then find the meals that best suit your body type.

If you're curious about the science supporting what we'll be doing and learning the "how" behind the "what do I eat," though, enjoy the chapters that follow.

It is important that you become familiar with what we will be doing. The better you understand the basics of the Body Type Diet, the easier it will be.

Can food combining really help you?

Everything you eat—destined to be broken down chemically and affect our bodies in one way or another—either helps you or hurts you.

When you first cut calories in an effort to lose weight, your body—a human fat-storing machine fixated on avoiding starvation—will initially allow for this calorie reduction. Once it recognizes it's no longer receiving either adequate nutrients or calories, though, its natural defense mechanisms, in an instinctual effort to protect itself and you from starvation, kick in and stubbornly cling to all future calories and food intake. In other words, you begin to store more and burn less. The human body also has a built-in mechanism called a fat set point, which is like a thermostat that regulates the temperature in a room. It therefore makes sense to feed your body not only a enough calories, but also the right nutrients in the right food combinations, as well. Satisfied it's getting enough food to survive; your body will then allow you to lose weight and get lean by helping you create a super-fast metabolism helping you burn more calories safely.

Remember, the body reacts to food.

For example, when you eat protein, your body gets "tighter." Why? Because protein draws water out of the body. Carbohydrates, on the other hand, draw water into the body. How does your body react? It makes you "softer." As you begin, you will see firsthand the dramatic effect certain foods in certain combinations can have on how you look and feel.

Some people have even found an improvement in their health. I've discovered that finding the right food combinations for my clients who struggle with issues such as diabetes or high cholesterol often results in a favorable, sometimes immediate impact on their bloodwork and over time helps them lead healthier, more comfortable lives.

What makes The Body Type Diet different?

1. Other diets focus on weight loss, but more important is body composition, the distribution of that weight. Fat weight versus lean weight. You can be down several sizes in clothing and still be the same weight.

2. Other diets emphasize calories. What is of more importance is nutrient ratios. How many grams of protein, fats, and carbohydrates am I getting? You can have 500 calories of fish or 500 calories of pizza, but one will get you lean and one will get you fat.

3. Other diets say that calories in versus calories out equals weight loss, which is not always true. Using a mathematical approach, if I cut 1,200 calories a day from my food intake, it will add up to 8,400 calories a week. Scientifically speaking there are 3,500 calories in a pound, so cutting 1,200 calories a day would create a weight loss of two to three pounds a week. If I typically eat 3,000 calories a day and change so that I eat 1,000 calories, I would be creating a 730,000-calorie deficit in a year, which would mean I could lose 200 pounds in a year and would weigh zero. I guess I would disappear.

4. Getting lean is what you want to do. Muscle is active; fat is inactive. One pound of lean tissue can burn fifty calorie a day, which is why you can keep the weight off by getting lean. By becoming leaner you increase your basal metabolic rate, the

number of calories your body burns at rest. Therefore, you will be able not only to lose weight but also keep it off, because your body is now burning more calories at rest. Many people who do not exercise still get lean and keep weight off. We do not exercise to lose weight. We exercise to improve our cardio-vascular health, create a euphoric state, and tighten and tone our bodies.

5. You must regulate four key hormones in regard to nutrition, insulin, glucagon, cortisol, and human growth hormone. If you don't regulate these hormones, you won't get anywhere. So how do you do that? By changing your meals frequently, by changing the times you eat, and changing the food combinations.

6. Fat burns in the flame of carbohydrates. You must have carbohydrates present in your body to trigger a fat-burning response. It is also important to note that carbohydrates allow for proper amino acid uptake into muscle cells to help with proper fluid placement. Remember water goes in only one of two places: inside a cell or outside a cell. We want it inside the cell, making us tight and firm.

7. The ultimate weight-loss formula is to get lean, decrease body fat, and lose water weight through lean-tissue development.

8. You need proper fluid placement and healthy electrolyte levels, better salt and sugar balance.

9. It is very important to note the biochemical breakdown of food on the body. When we eat something, how is that food broken down? On my plan you can eat many foods that you thought where making you fat, only to find out those foods are now making you lose fat. Such foods include dark chocolate, peanut butter, and cream cheese.

10. It's not just about eating healthy foods. Many of us do eat healthy foods. Losing weight is about eating correctly, which is where food combining becomes important. Here is a great

example: a client comes to me with diabetes. We go over the person's nutrition plan, and I find the client is already eating healthy foods. Three months later the client no longer has diabetes. Here is how I changed things:

	Their way	Body Type Diet way
Meal 1	bowl of oatmeal, raisins, and berries	oatmeal plus 3 egg whites
Meal 2	fruit salad	fruit salad plus 20 almonds
Meal 3	turkey on whole wheat and apple	turkey on whole wheat with cucumber
Meal 4	beans, potato, chicken	chicken, green veggies, potato
After dinner	rice cakes and jelly	rice cakes with jelly and peanut butter

The client was making healthy choices but not eating correctly. All the foods the client was eating were turning to sugar in the bloodstream and causing high blood-sugar levels. Here is what we learned. The client was making healthy food choices, but all the carbohydrates eaten together without sufficient protein or fat was turning to sugar and then turning to fat.

- With meal 1, I added the egg whites as the protein source. By adding protein you are able to process the sugar from the oatmeal and get lean.
- With meal 2, the fruit salad by itself was turning to sugar and actually making this person very lethargic. By adding a good source of fat from the almonds you are able to process the sugar and actually increase your energy.
- With meal 3, I took out the apple because the carbohydrates

from the bread were plenty; the apple added too many carbohydrates, which again turned to sugar. Taking out the apple and adding cucumber helped the body get rid of extra salt and sugar, because cucumber acts as a natural diuretic.

- With meal 4, the beans and potato are a carbohydrate plus a carbohydrate, which turns to double sugar and double fat. I took out the beans and added some cleansing green vegetables.

- With the after-dinner meal, rice cakes and jelly is sugar plus sugar again. We need some type of protein or fat to help process the sugar, so I added peanut butter.

What are we really trying to do?

The real science of the Body Type Diet lies not only in eating the right foods for your body, but in getting lean. Getting lean is important.

Lean simply indicates that the muscle cell is drawing in more water, thereby tightening the texture of your skin. The more lean muscle you have—because muscle is active, while fat is inactive—the more calories you burn. In fact you burn more—even without exercise—for long periods of time, the leaner you are. Getting you lean is therefore one of our first goals, but don't worry. Gaining lean muscle does not equal being big and muscular. Lean is a good thing. One pound of lean muscle can not only burn up to sixty calories a day but also carry up to two pounds of water between the cells.

Our aim is to help your body burn more calories, whether you're sitting at a desk, behind the wheel of your car, or just going on about your day. Regardless of how you spend your time, I want you to stay lean and keep the weight off. But how is that achieved?

By altering your body composition and increasing your BMR.

Everyone has what we call a basal metabolic rate (or BMR), an indicator of how many calories your body burns at rest. One of the most effective methods for losing weight and keeping it off is by increasing this BMR. Altering your body composition—in other words—becoming leaner and decreasing your body fat—is one of the best ways of stepping up your BMR, helping you burn more calories at rest.

But any good program such as the Body Type Diet must take into account the type of weight being lost, and you want it to be the "right weight."

When we first increase your lean weight, you'll find yourself holding temporary water weight. Don't panic. Before you know it, we'll be decreasing your body fat, which will help you quickly lose the temporary water weight and then the weight from fat. More importantly, the weight you will be losing will be composed of excess water, salt and sugar. It'll be the "right weight."

Now that you have a better understanding of what The Body Type Diet is, let's start talking about food and the human body.

The Human Body

Everything in your body exists and works solely for one purpose: to keep you alive and healthy. And it is only through the food you eat in its three basic forms—carbohydrates, protein, and fat—that the body is able to do this.

But just what are carbohydrates, protein, and fat?

Generally, carbohydrates exist in the form of sugar, while fat is found in the various forms of lecithin, cholesterol, or triglycerides.

Protein—the predominant nutrient in The Body Type Diet—is very different, however. While there are only a few forms of fats and carbohydrates, there are thousands of recognized forms of protein. In fact, 75% of your body—enzymes, cells, hormones, muscles, and tissues—is made up of protein. This overwhelming number of protein structures is the reason behind everyone being physiologically different.

The protein you eat is first broken up into smaller constituents called amino acids and then reconstructed to meet your body's needs. What makes food combining so effective is the way these amino acid "building blocks" link together before being broken down in the body.

The successful functioning of your body is dependent on amino acids. How they are used and which metabolic pathway—a map that charts the direction nutrients take once ingested in your body—is chosen depends on the body's needs at that time as well as whether or not the food was eaten in the correct combination.

Health imbalances can result if there is a shortage of amino acids, with the whole body being affected by a single minor deficiency. The body operates so precisely that if the right nutrients aren't present, you cannot properly digest your food, making it difficult to absorb what you need from what you eat adequately. This unfortunately will result in the continuous depletion of amino acids, causing not only a drop in hormone production, but also a dramatically limited number of amino acids available for protein synthesis. And without protein synthesis, the body won't be able to build lean muscle and burn calories.

In addition, because of this lack of proper nutrients, your body will find itself with less insulin to regulate blood sugar levels, not enough adrenaline to deal with stress, and a decrease in thyroxin, a thyroid-secreting hormone that effectively works with metabolism and the immune system. A body struggling in these conditions will eventually find itself battling disease and illness.

A great deal of what I give you with food combinations in The Body Type Diet is designed to strengthen the innate metabolic reactions in your body naturally, helping you not only to look great, but also feel good and stay healthy.

Chapter 2

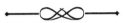

Why It Works: The Body Type Fundamentals

You are finally going to lose the weight and keep it off. How will it happen? By following a specific nutritional plan for your body type. As you have already learned, we all have our own unique genetic makeup, so it makes no sense for us all to eat the same way. The Body Type Diet will become a new way of life for you. It is a way of making nutrition a healthy, integral part of your daily life. By committing to this program and understanding its fundamentals, you will lose the weight.

The foods that form the basis of The Body Type Diet are animal proteins, whey protein, grains, beans, fruits, and vegetables. The Body Type Diet is a balanced eating plan with a specific and ample supply of nutrients that are required by your specific body-type needs. It also moderates unwanted fats, such as hydrogenated fats and trans fats, as well as sugars and salts.

The Body Type Diet meals are successful because of the following:

1. They are high in amino acid values, the building blocks of protein and muscle tissue. Amino acids are very important because they enable our bodies to become leaner.

2. They have high nutrient density, the measure of nutrients provided per calorie of food.
3. They have a high thermic effect; they raise your metabolism.
4. They have lower energy density; they can quickly be digested and absorbed and leave your body at a faster rate.

Today people choose the foods they feel are good for them based on 1) what they read and learn from diet books, 2) literature and/or advertisements, 3) convenience and affordability, or 4) because of their cultural traditions. While the United States Department of Health and Human Services sets health objectives for the nation and monitors our nutritional status, it is a well-known fact that an increasing number of adults and children are not meeting nutritional goals for healthy living. Although the nation is striving for balance and moderation by eating the correct foods, according to the US Department of Health and Human Services, "currently only 1% of the population achieves these elements at the same time." With the knowledge you're learning in this book, you are going to be part of a majority that is in control.

The Three Fundamentals behind The Body Type Diet

The main reason this program works so effectively and efficiently is because you are eating meals specifically designed for your body type. Food either helps us or hurts us; it is not neutral. It can either be burned as calories or stored in the body as fat. What follows is a closer look at the fundamentals of The Body Type Diet. If you remember to incorporate these fundamentals, you will succeed.

FUNDAMENTAL NUMBER ONE: LOSING WEIGHT THE RIGHT WAY

I cannot stress this enough: if you want to lose weight and keep weight off, you need to become lean. When you are lean your body burns more calories, more efficiently. If you build more lean tissue, your body will burn more calories at rest. This process is referred to as your basal metabolic rate (BMR). By getting leaner, you are burning more calories at rest, which allows you to keep the weight off, even without exercise.

When most people think of weight loss, they think of it as the number they see on the scale, but the scale indicates only your actual weight, not the distribution of that weight. The scale does not tell you the composition of that weight, and it is body composition that matters most. You want to know what percentage of you is lean and what percentage of you is fat. If you are worried only about the weight—that pesky number—you will lose muscle, which is what burns calories. You will also be making your metabolism less efficient. If you want to lose weight, look and feel great, and keep weight off, you have to understand body composition. It is quite possible to lose body fat, get leaner, lose inches, and experience only a small weight loss, which is what you see in the two photos of me at the same weight—lean mass versus fat mass.

What you are learning to do with The Body Type Diet is enable your body to perform better by working with its natural mechanisms.

Losing weight the right way is one fundamental. Let's move on to the second one.

FUNDAMENTAL NUMBER TWO: CREATING A FAST METABOLISM

One of the main goals of The Body Type Diet is to help you lose weight and lose body fat. This is achieved by having your body burn more calories all the time.

Whether you are active or at rest you want your body to burn calories and create a faster, more efficient metabolism. Feeding your body every two to three hours facilitates a faster, more efficient metabolism. It is essential not to miss meals or skip meals because this will slow down your metabolism. If you are not hungry, it's permissible to skip a meal, just remember to drink plenty of water. If you happen to get hungry before your next meal, I provided you with specific "if hungry choices" on your Body Type meal plan. If you feel hungry at times, this is a good thing; it is your body telling you that it is hard at work burning fat. Feeding it will enable your body to burn more fat and lose more weight.

Many clients have reported that after following The Body Type Diet they went from never being hungry to always being hungry. This is because we have ignited your metabolism and it is working in a faster mode.

There is nothing wrong with being hungry. The important thing is to make healthier choices to satisfy this sensation, not fast food.

Over the years I have found that the times of day we eat are relatively 9am, 12pm, 3pm, 5pm and 7-8pm. Therefore, I decided five to be the best number of meals to eat while on The Body Type Diet. If you eat too many meals too soon your body cannot digest all the food you have eaten. If you go long periods without eating your metabolism will slow down. Remember, it takes the body about two to three hours to digest and process all its nutrients.

What's great about The Body Type Diet is that your body begins working more efficiently. Then food you eat that was once being stored as body fat is now being burned as fuel. By eating every few hours, you are providing your body with the right amounts of nutrients, specifically protein, to help you become leaner.

Remember, you really can't get lean and lose weight by eating three square meals. Before coming to me, almost every one of my overweight clients had been eating three meals day and it was not working.

Another great thing about eating small frequent meals is that your blood sugar levels become more stable, you will have more energy and you will not be prone to craving bad, non-nutritional food. Over the years, many clients have told me they no longer crave junk food. This is because your body is happy and satisfied; it has the correct nutrients so it can perform efficiently. They also tell me if they eat junk food they feel sick. This is because your blood is so clean and it reacts adversely to anything unclean. You also need to know that protein, composed of the powerful amino acids we need, remains in the bloodstream for about two to three hours; then you need more protein. Thus, small frequent meals spread throughout the day will lead to a faster metabolism.

Now on the weekends we might be a little off of our schedule and that's okay. Just think about what you are doing and what your objective is—to lose weight the correct way. It's acceptable to cheat every now and then, but with The Body Type Diet it's easy to get back on track. Let's use me for an example. Because my body fat levels are low, I can occasionally eat junk food and burn it at high levels. This is very important for you to remember because this will allow you to indulge once in a while.

It is habit forming because it is easy and it works.

Having a fast metabolism is the second fundamental for maximum weight loss. Let's move on to the final fundamental.

FUNDAMENTAL NUMBER THREE: COMBINING FOOD FOR OPTIMAL RESULTS

The Body Type Diet meals consist of properly combined foods that work best for your body type. These combinations produce an important effect on your body when eaten together and ultimately give you the body you desire. These food combinations more successfully stimulate weight loss and improve the quality of your health.

When you follow The Body Type Diet you reduce your sugar and sodium (salt) intake. Numerous studies have concluded that excess sugar and sodium cause weight gain and can lead to diseases and complications such as diabetes, high cholesterol, hypoglycemia, and obesity.

The Body Type Diet integrates the basic principle of sugar reduction; however, I've found that excess sodium is just as bad for you. You may notice that when you eat a lot of salt your body looks and feels bloated. The reason is that salt attracts water and turns your body into a sponge. What causes the bloating is the location of salt accumulation in your body—just beneath your skin, in the subcutaneous tissue, rather than inside your muscle cells.

I like to use the slug as an example. A slug, like your cells, is composed mainly of water. Imagine what happens when you put salt on the slug. All the water gets drawn out of the slug, and it shrivels up. Another good example is for all you cooks out there. What do you do when you are preparing eggplant? You put salt on a slice of eggplant to draw out the water.

The subcutaneous layer beneath your skin has a major influence on your appearance. You may be thinking that this is simple—that all you have to do is cut down your sodium intake, thereby reducing the amount of water that is drawn out of the cells. Well, you are only partially right.

The second part involves drawing water into the muscle cells. How? By increasing your potassium intake. Potassium is like sodium; in fact they both attract water. However, potassium, unlike sodium, is found in the muscle cells. By drawing water into the muscle cells, the subcutaneous tissue beneath your skin shrinks, and you lose that bloated look. On the Body Type Diet you will lose weight, your body composition will change, and you will have better water placement inside the cells. Your lean weight will increase and your fat weight will decrease. The Body Type Diet food combining consists of maintaining the proper sodium/potassium ratios or electrolyte (mineral) balance.

The main reasons The Body Type Meal Combinations are so successful for weight loss include the following:

1. You are able to maintain a positive nitrogen balance state, which means that the body receives all the protein it needs, so it can do its job of building lean tissue, burning fat, and losing weight. You will therefore notice that almost every meal combination contains a protein. If you are not meeting your protein requirements, your muscles will atrophy, you will store calories instead of burning them, and your body will take protein from the reserve tank found in your blood-protein levels. Remember, you must keep protein constant at every meal, because if you eat only carbohydrates, you lose the chemical reactions that make food burn more efficiently. A food without a protein requires that your body must break down muscle to get the amino acids it needs. What most people are doing on a diet is eating their own muscle. Remember, one pound of lean tissue burns about fifty calories a day so focus on becoming leaner, and you will lose more weight.

2. You are able to get the proteins and amino acids into the muscle cells so they can do their job and you can experience that tight, toned feeling. For this to happen the body needs insulin, which is produced when we eat carbohydrates. Therefore, a moderate amount of carbohydrates with each meal is important to support the amino acid uptake into the muscle cells.

3. Eating carbohydrates by themselves is like shooting sugar into the bloodstream. You really don't want to eat carbohydrates alone, so fruit by itself is not a good idea. You need some good fat to burn the sugar from the fruit. Some good fats can be found in cheese and nuts, so if you have twelve almonds and an apple, it automatically becomes a fat-burning meal because of the omega 3 good fats (the almonds) mixed with the carbohydrates (the apple).

4. You learn food combinations that give you a slow release of insulin into the bloodstream. High insulin secretions promote higher body fat storage and increase your weight. For example, the sports performance meal combination of graham crackers and turkey or graham crackers and peanut butter and jelly provides a slow release of insulin because peanut butter and turkey contain adequate amino acids. These amino acids help the body produce more lean tissue as a result of their chemical nature.

5. Because of the food combinations' amino acid content and profiles, they allow for sustained energy and lower blood sugar levels. It is important to provide your body with essential and nonessential amino acids. Some your body makes, and some your body doesn't, but you need both, to become lean.

6. I have developed custom-blend protein shakes for each body type. The blend consists of the right amino acids to help you get lean and burn fat.

Chapter 3

————∞————

Determining
Your Body Type

Body Type is a term used to describe the percentage of fat to lean muscle mass. We also call it body composition—in other words, the distribution of your weight. Simply put, how many pounds are lean and how many pounds are fat? Because of the connection between Body Type and how our bodies process food, I have established four body types. Each Body Type is based on sound science, and one of the types will fit you.

For as long as I have been studying and teaching nutrition I have always said, "Your body is the most important thing in life." Without your body functioning in a healthy manner, and without feeling good about your body, it is very hard to live a completely stress-free life. If you can take control of your body and health, you can do just about anything you want in life. I am going to show you what thousands of others have already experienced, the power to change the way you look and feel by investing just a few minutes of time each day.

The questionnaire is a very simple method for identifying your Body Type and finding what specific meals work with your Body Type. It will take approximately five minutes. Read each question carefully and circle the answer that best describes you right now. Take your time and remember, there are no right and wrong answers—only positive feedback.

The test will ask you twenty questions about your metabolism and twenty questions about your body composition, all of which are vital for determining your Body Type. The test, which is based on my research over the past twelve years, incorporates data I compiled on clients' weight loss, weight kept off, composition change, and overall bloodwork health. I have studied how various foods, when present in the right combinations, affected clients' results. I even compared clients' results based on those who exercised and those who did not. My amazing discovery? Nutrition was about 80% of the formula.

With all this talk about body type, the power of amino acids, and the success of building lean muscle has on burning calories, you're probably wondering "Well, when do we begin?"

We'll start by identifying your body type with a questionnaire I've developed—The Body Type Test. From there we can then move to the specific foods best suited for your body type enabling you not only to lose weight, but also keep it off.

Get a pencil and some paper, and let's begin the part that's fun.

Putting Your Body Type to the Test

Answer the following forty questions.

1. Take the number that is most common after you have answered each question. That predominant number determines your body type.
2. Here is an example: 1211434111122243111111111245111 1112111111. In this case, you would be a bloated fat body type, because you have twenty-seven number ones.

Once you finish the questionnaire, you'll know which of the four body types you have, and then you can move directly into the next chapters, in which you'll learn which foods work best with your body type. You will be on your way to losing weight and feeling better than you ever have before.

Here's to your success!

Twenty Questions about Your Metabolism

1. My body is responsive to salt and sugar
    1. extremely
    2. moderately
    3. a little
    4. cannot tell

2. How many meals a day do you eat?
    1. more than 5
    2. 3 to 5
    3. varies
    4. not many, but long gaps in between

3. After eating carbohydrates, I feel
    1. tired and sluggish
    2. very soft
    3. solid
    4. happy and satisfied (or cannot tell)

4. On average, I drink this many 8-ounce glasses of water a day
    1. 0 to 3
    2. 3 to 6
    3. 6 to 8
    4. more than 8

5. I exercise
    1. not at all
    2. 3 to 5 times a week
    3. daily
    4. excessively (more than once a day)

6. I drink soda
    1. 5 to 10 times a week
    2. 3 to 5 times a week
    3. all the time
    4. not much or not at all

7. I can eat anything and I
    1. gain lots of weight
    2. don't gain much weight, I just get softer
    3. find my weight fluctuates
    4. find my weight stays the same

8. I barely eat, and I
    1. gain weight
    2. experience very little weight change but feel softer
    3. notice that my weight fluctuates
    4. stay at the same weight

9. I have always been fit, but lately my body is
    1. unfit
    2. very responsive to exercise
    3. not responding
    4. only somewhat responsive to exercise

10. Generally speaking I
    1. have struggled with weight all my life
    2. have alternated between periods of fit and fat
    3. gain weight quickly
    4. maintain the same weight

11. Physically speaking
    1. I tire easy
    2. I have stages of energy and no energy
    3. I am fairly athletic despite my layer of fat
    4. I am fairly active

12. I sleep
    1. more than 8 hours
    2. 8 hours
    3. 5 to 6 hours
    4. 4 hours or less: do not really require a lot of sleep

13. If I don't eat for a while
    1. I am fine
    2. I eat moderately
    3. I become ravenous
    4. I binge big time

14. I have tried the following diets over the years
    1. every one of them
    2. only a few
    3. Atkins and other higher protein, higher fat diets
    4. None

15. I eat late
    1. every night
    2. more than once a night
    3. only occasionally at night
    (4.) I don't really eat late at night

16. Food to me
    1. consumes my life
    2. is very comforting
    3. is energy
    (4.) is no big deal

17. I drink alcohol
    1. 5 or more drinks a week
    2. 3 to 5 drinks a week
    3. 3 drinks or less a week
    (4.) do not drink

18. My current health status is
    1. diabetes, high cholesterol, obesity; serious health problems
    2. minor health issues
    (3.) high cholesterol and/or diabetes
    4. pretty healthy

19. After I eat I
    1. cannot wait to eat again
    2. feel tired
    (3.) feel satisfied
    4. am always hungry

20. I can look at food and
    1. I gain weight
    2. I binge
    3. I get excited
    4. I have no real feelings toward food

Good job. Stay focused! We are almost finished.

The next twenty questions are about your body composition.

1. I prefer salt or sugar
    1. both
    2. both, but more sugar
    3. both, but more salt
    4. neither

2. My morning weight and evening weight is
    1. always drastically different
    2. a 2- to 4-pound difference
    3. high both times
    4. not much change or cannot tell

3. I gain most of my weight
    1. midsection, hips, and buttocks
    2. midsection
    3. everywhere
    4. not much weight difference, just get softer

4. I eat junk food
    1. 5 or more times a week
    2. 3 to 5 times a week
    3. occasionally
    4. never

5. I eat fried foods
    1. 5 or more times a week
    (2.) fewer than 5 times a week
    3. all the time
    4. not too often or never

6. My current energy levels are
    1. extremely low
    (2.) high and low
    3. high
    4. normal

7. When I exercise, I lose weight
    1. fast
    2. moderately
    3. very slowly
    (4.) do not lose weight

8. If I am stressed, I will often resort to
    1. candy bars
    2. pasta or bread
    3. chips, soda, and junk foods
    (4.) granola, nuts, or do not eat

9. If I had to describe my body, I would say I am
    1. obese
    (2.) overweight
    3. big and solid
    4. very soft

10. I used to look great and now I
    1. never looked great to begin with
    2. cannot recognize my body
    3. have a layer of fat covering me
    4. feel soft

11. I have had trouble with my weight
    1. all my life
    2. been up and down over the years
    3. for the past 5 to 10 years
    4. for the past few years or more recently

12. In addition to being overweight, I have
    1. a great deal of water retention
    2. little shape and definition
    3. high body fat
    4. a very soft feeling

13. If I make a muscle, I feel
    1. soft
    2. tight
    3. hard
    4. lean

14. Which part of your body gains weight the fastest?
    1. stomach
    2. love handles and midsection
    3. entire body
    4. arms and skin gain weight and get flabby

15. My weight is affecting
    1. my entire life
    (2) some areas of my life
    3. not really affecting me, but I would like to lose some weight
    4. not really affecting me, but I want better body composition

16. Currently I feel
    1. 50 pounds or more overweight
    (2.) 5 to 20 pounds overweight
    3. 25 to 50 pounds overweight
    4. 5 to 10 pounds overweight. It's not really about weight; it is more about better body composition

17. If I lost all my fat, I would be
    1. smaller
    (2) defined
    3. athletic
    4. lean

18. What runs in my family?
    1. Obesity, a great deal
    (2) Being overweight
    3. High amounts of body fat
    4. None of these run in my family

19. People look at me
    1. in a strange way
    (2) normally
    3. as a fat person
    4. cannot tell

20. If I lost all my weight my life would be
    1. incredible
    2. a little better
    ③ healthier
    4. the same

Fantastic! Great job! Now you can see your predominate number and apply it to the body types explained in the next chapter, so you can learn how to eat correctly to lose weight and finally keep it off.

Okay, now I am going to explain to you the four different body types and the characteristics that make up each type. Once you learn more about your body type and the meals that go with your body type, you can then go right to your eating plan.

Chapter 4

———∞———

The Four Body Types

Biochemical characteristics are unique to each person. I learned through my twenty-five years dealing with thousands of clients that people could be classified into four different body types, thereby giving each type a customized nutritional plan. Here are the four body types:

Body Type 1, Bloated Fat

Your body type experiences a major reaction in terms of your skin being swollen and puffy. Your body type reacts to both salts and sugars. Your weight tends to develop from ingesting too much salt, sugar, and carbohydrates and not enough protein. Your type can experience dramatic fluctuations in weight, and bloated types are usually those who are overweight and obese. You may have been chubby as a child.

BODY COMPOSITION
- Your body is large and round
- You seem to be large in your midsection and waist
- You have more fat weight compared to your lean weight
- Your muscles are not well developed
- Your body is soft and puffy

METABOLISM
- You have very slow metabolism
- Much of the food you eat tends to add weight quickly
- It is hard for you to lose weight

Body Type 2, Soft Fat

This body type experiences a major reaction in terms of the skin being very soft. Often soft fat people have a difficult time breaking down carbohydrates, especially breads, pasta, and fruit. They tend to be insulin resistant, which means when sugar is ingested it remains in their bloodstream and quickly turns to fat. Because these carbohydrates and sugars are lingering in their body, their skin tends to soften up.

COMPOSITION
- Your shape is like a block, very square
- You have good lean muscle mass beneath your soft covering
- You tend to gain weight in your midsection and grow love handles
- Your body tends to soften up very quickly
- Your body type can be very fit or very fat

METABOLISM
- Your body is very responsive to exercise
- You gain fat weight easily
- Your metabolism is slow
- You can build lean muscle mass very quickly and can maintain it well

Body Type 3, Solid Fat

This body type experiences a major reaction in terms of the skin being very solid and firm, but solid and firm from too much fat. Often solid fat people have a difficult time breaking down fats. The fat they ingest lingers in their body and can even cause a high volume of triglycerides in the blood. Triglycerides are our body's stored fat. Solid Fat body types have usually eaten a great deal of fat or have tried high-fat diets over the years.

COMPOSITION

- Your body type is very thick
- There is a great deal of fat covering your lean muscle mass
- Your body texture is tight with a high amount of body fat

METABOLISM

- Your metabolism is not that slow
- You tend not to gain much weight, but rather gain more body fat
- You build and maintain lean muscle mass very easily.

Body Type 4, Skinny Fat

This body type experiences a major reaction in terms of the skin being soft and mushy. Often skinny fat body types are more prevalent with females because much has to do with hormonal irregularities. Skinny fat people also have a difficult time breaking down nutrients. Skinny fat types also have a difficult time getting lean. Their bodies tend to be smaller and have a high body fat percentage. Did you ever see a skinny guy with a big stomach, a gut or beer belly? This is a skinny fat type. Many younger females tend to develop what I call a pouch; the lower portion of their stomach is swollen.

This skinny fat type is also prevalent in women going through menopause. These abnormalities tend to develop from hormonal irregularities and not eating the right foods. Often these skinny fat types eat bananas, whole grains, granola, and hummus, many foods that are high in carbohydrates and very low in protein, and because of the lack of protein, skinny fat types soften right up. Without the presence of high-quality protein, the foods they are eating are being stored as fat rather than being burned as fuel.

COMPOSITION
- Your body type may have been lean at one point, but over time you lost a great deal of muscle mass
- You have more fat weight than lean weight
- Your frame tends to be smaller

METABOLISM
- Your metabolism is fast, but so fast, you can lose lean muscle mass quickly
- Your body burns calories quickly and you tend to appear soft looking
- You experience major hormonal fluctuations

Chapter 5

———∞———

High-Powered Body Type Meals

Okay, this is where the real fun begins and what really separates The Body Type Diet from every other diet on the market. Let me recap what most diets provide you with. They consist of tricks so you lose water weight and a menu of foods to eat that are lower in calories, with the hope that if you take in fewer calories than you burn, you will lose weight.

Here is what you've learned so far. You've learned there are four body types, and each body type responds best to certain combinations of meals. The powerful and dynamic breakdown of these food combinations and categories of meals triggers a body fat and weight reduction response.

The reason these meal combinations are so effective is that they are customized for your specific body type. This information is what you will be using to design your meal programs.

The key to your Body Type Meals is not just the individual foods you'll choose but the combination of foods you select and arrange into meals. Let's be honest. None of us can simply eat whatever we want whenever we want and actually expect to live a long, healthy life. Good nutrition and health are things we must work to achieve and maintain.

And it's not all about just eating healthy foods. These days food no longer exists in its natural state. Chemicals, additives, preservatives, and fillers have made their way into our food. which is why the use of proper food combining is crucial to achieve balance and provide the body with materials and chemicals that cells need to perform their task of tissue repair, muscle growth, and sustaining good health and high energy levels.

With that said, let's get into the two specific meal categories for each body type and the two interchangeable meals for everyone.

Body Type 1, Bloated Fat Meals

1. Water-Balance Meals
    - Water-balance meals are designed to draw excess water out of your body. The natural process of getting lean means the body is initially going to hold onto water. These meals help rid the body of the excess water that we tend to carry in our intestines where you really do not want much water weight. An example of a water-balance meal is cheese and grapes.

2. Weight-Loss Meals
    - Weight-loss meals have what we call lower-energy-density foods, meaning the combinations of foods you eat enter your body, do their job, and leave rather quickly. They also tend to produce a higher thermic effect, which will in effect speed up your metabolism and help you burn more calories at a faster rate. The thermic effect of a meal is the energy that takes place after you eat a meal containing the body's key nutrients. An example of a weight-loss meal is Raisin Bran cereal and a slice of cheese or a Blend Shape protein shake.

Body Type 2: Soft Fat Meals

1. Sports-Performance Meals
    *   Sports-performance meals refers to a category of food that contains the greatest amount of protein and all the essential and nonessential amino acids required to get your body lean. These meals also help increase your BMR, which refers to the number of calories you burn at rest, so you will burn more calories around the clock, even without exercise. An example of a sports-performance meal is egg whites and oatmeal or a Lean Blend protein shake.

2. Complete Athlete Meals
    *   Complete athlete meals are like sports-performance meals, except that they have more of a lean mass stimulator amino acid called N-acetylcysteine, to prevent your body from losing any lean weight. As you age your body naturally loses lean mass over time; so complete athlete meals keep us from breaking down our lean mass. These meals also contain a little more carbohydrates to help draw more water into your muscle cells, keeping you tighter and firmer for longer periods. An example of a complete athlete meal is egg whites, turkey, and potato or a Blend Athlete protein shake.

Body Type 3: Solid Fat Meals

1. Fat-Burning Meals
    *   Fat-burning meals not only speed up your metabolism and help your body burn fat more quickly, but also contain foods that have a lower glycemic index. The glycemic index indicates how much and how fast sugar hits your bloodstream. If food has a high glycemic index, it will lead to more fat weight and fat storage. With these meals you

will inhibit your body from packing on the pounds. In fact, eating lower glycemic meals may be healthier for you because of the stabilization of insulin levels and a possible decreased risk of heart conditions. Fat-burning meals also promote lower body fat levels and a leaner physique, allowing for only small rises in blood sugar levels, which can help control diabetes or improve your blood-sugar metabolism. An example of a fat-burning meal is an apple and yogurt or a Blend Melt protein shake.

2. Thermogenic Meals
    *   Similar to fat-burning meals, thermogenic meals actually help your body produce a thermogenic response. What it means is that your body burns calories as heat, and at times you will feel your body getting hot and sweaty, which means your body is in a thermogenic mode. An example of a thermogenic meal is red pepper and cottage cheese or Blend Shape or Melt protein shake.

Body Type 4, Skinny Fat Meals

1. Hormonal-Balance Meals
    *   You've heard of women, weight, and hormones. Well, hormonal-balance meals actually help your body regulate hormones more efficiently. Sometimes women can carry little tummy pouches and men little potbellies, often due to hormonal imbalances. The many changing hormone levels in their bodies need to be regulated better. An example of a hormonal-balance meal is pretzels and cream cheese or Blend Nourish protein shake.
2. Tone 'n' Tighten Meals
    *   Tone 'n' tighten meals help balance your electrolyte levels. Electrolytes are key minerals in the body that help give you proper fluid placement. If you want to be tight and firm,

tone 'n' tighten meals will do the trick. Many times we eat carbohydrates, and they tend to linger in our bodies and attract water accumulation. These meals help draw fluid inside the cell so your skin actually gets tighter. An example of a tone 'n' tighten meal is peanut butter and jelly on multigrain bread or Blend Tighten supplement with lemon.

Two Interchangeable Meals for all Body Types

1. Basic Nutrient Meals
    *   Basic nutrient meals contain the proper balance of proteins, carbohydrates, and fat. They can be eaten as a replacement meal for any of your specified body type meals at any time. These meals also have a little more fiber to help your body process food better. An example of a basic nutrient meal is chicken, salad, asparagus, and brown rice.
2. Salt and Sugar Meals
    *   Salt and sugar meals contain a combination of salt and sugar and provide your body with a proper ratio of minerals. Minerals are very important with respect to the proper fluid placement in your body. These meals can also be eaten as a replacement meal for any of your specified body type meals at any time. An example of a salt and sugar meal is almonds and an orange.

Chapter 6

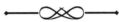

Customized Eating Plans for Fast Results

Using the Plans—How They Work

You are going to learn how to lose weight and keep it off by using one of the four customized food plans that are tailored to your specific body type. I know you have been through many diets and have tried desperately to lose weight. With these food plans, backed by sound science, you will now do just that—lose weight. All you have to do is check your scale and watch the pounds melt off.

Please make sure you correctly identify your body type and eating plan before you begin. By now you should know all the fundamentals to eating correctly for your body type. Eat from the specific meal categories for your body type and remember you can always choose the two listed interchangeable meals any time (basic nutrient meal and salt and sugar meals), regardless of your body type.

I have provided you with plenty of choices. Your menu consists of five meals a day. You can choose what to eat anytime between your meals, but only if you feel hungry.

Please remember the following:

- Try not to miss meals.

- Drink plenty of water, especially if you skip a meal because you're not hungry.
- Use your replacement meals for any meal once a day, as they add variety.
- Use condiments sparingly. You can always add three teaspoons of low-fat dressings to your salads. Condiments and dressings are fine because your fat, salt and sugar intake is relatively low and the condiments will be burned more readily.
- Enjoy the process.

Here's how it works:

Turn to the meal template for your body type. Follow the menu for the week. It is important to alternate between the meal categories each week. For example, let's say you are a Body Type 2, soft fat. Week 1 you want to choose sports-performance meals, and week two you want to choose complete athlete meals, and then repeat the process, so week 3 is back to sports-performance meals. You can always add any of the two interchangeable meals of salt and sugar and basic nutrient for any of your meals. Please keep in mind the more variety you choose initially, the more you will help your hormones become regulated better and the more results you will achieve. Once you reach your ideal target weight, you can eat more of the same foods, and they will help you maintain your results.

The Food Plans for Each Body Type

Body Type 1, Bloated Fat

Your body type is one that is very responsive to salt and sugar. A great deal of the foods you have been eating contained abundant amounts of salt and sugar that caused water retention and excess weight gain. Sodium makes you retain excess water weight, and sugar causes an increase in your insulin levels, which leads to weight gain.

The meals you will be eating are weight-loss and water-balance meals that specifically target your body type. These meals are very powerful and will help your body rid itself of excess salt and sugar and help you become leaner.

It is best to choose two weight-loss meals and two water-balance meals. The additional meal can be either another weight-loss meal, water-balance meal, basic-nutrient meal, salt and sugar meal, or replacement meal.

Below is your meal plan for the week.

DAY-BY-DAY EATING PLAN FOR BODY TYPE 1, BLOATED FAT

MONDAY

Meal 1 Breakfast
Blend Melt protein shake

Meal 2 Lunch
6 oz. chicken/small tossed salad, and 1 apple

Meal 3 Snack
3 slices turkey and 15 almonds

Meal 4 Snack
8 oz. low-fat yogurt and 20 grapes

Meal 5 Dinner
4 egg-white omelet/2 slices low-fat cheese, and 1 cup pineapple

P.M. Snack (optional)
1 cup berries/4 tsp. peanut butter

DAY-BY-DAY EATING PLAN FOR BODY TYPE 1, BLOATED FAT

TUESDAY

Meal 1 Breakfast
4 egg whites and 1 pear

Meal 2 Lunch
4 slices turkey and sliced apple on whole wheat (2 slices)

Meal 3 Snack
6 oz. cottage cheese and 3 tbsp. sunflower seeds

Meal 4 Snack
20 almonds and 3 fig newtons

Meal 5 Dinner
8 oz. fresh fish and 1 cup cauliflower

P.M. Snack (optional)
2 rice cakes with 3 tsp. peanut butter and jelly

DAY-BY-DAY EATING PLAN FOR BODY TYPE 1, BLOATED FAT

WEDNESDAY

Meal 1 Breakfast

Melt or Shape Blend shake

Meal 2 Lunch

1 can tuna and 10 almonds and 1/2 cup brown rice

Meal 3 Snack

1 string cheese and 20 cashews

Meal 4 Snack

12 Wheat Thins and 3 slices turkey

Meal 5 Dinner

8 oz. turkey burger with 1 sweet potato and 1 cup greens

P.M. Snack (optional)

1 graham cracker with 4 tsp. peanut butter

DAY-BY-DAY EATING PLAN FOR BODY TYPE 1, BLOATED FAT

THURSDAY

Meal 1 Breakfast
Melt or Shape protein shake

Meal 2 Lunch
4 egg whites and 1 cup greens and 1 peach or pear

Meal 3 Snack
8 oz. yogurt and 20 cashews

Meal 4 Snack
15 almonds and 3 egg whites

Meal 5 Dinner
8 oz. chicken breast and ½ avocado in salad

P.M. Snack (optional)
20 grapes and 2 slices low-fat cheese

DAY-BY-DAY EATING PLAN FOR BODY TYPE 1, BLOATED FAT

FRIDAY

Meal 1 Breakfast

Melt or Shape protein shake

Meal 2 Lunch

1 can tuna on 2 slices rye and ½ cucumber

Meal 3 Snack

1 tomato and 1 apple

Meal 4 Snack

1 red pepper and 8 oz. cottage cheese

Meal 5 Dinner

4 egg omelet with cheese and veggies

P.M. Snack (optional)

1 cup granola and 8 oz. low-fat milk

Day-By-Day Eating Plan for Body Type 1, Bloated Fat
(with recipes)

Saturday

Meal 1 Breakfast
1 cup Kashi Golean cereal and 10 oz. low-fat milk and 10 almonds

Meal 2 Lunch
4 slices turkey and sliced tomato on whole grain (2 slices)

Meal 3 Snack
15 almonds and 2 pieces dark chocolate squares

Meal 4 Snack
8 oz. yogurt and 10 almonds and 10 cashews

Meal 5 Dinner
1 cup pasta and 8 oz. lean ground beef and tomato sauce

P.M. Snack (optional)
2 slices low-fat cheese and 10 grapes

DAY-BY-DAY EATING PLAN FOR BODY TYPE 1, BLOATED FAT
(WITH RECIPES)

SUNDAY

Meal 1 Breakfast
5 egg white omelet and 1 English muffin with 3 tsp. peanut butter

Meal 2 Lunch
2 cup greens and 8 oz. chicken

Meal 3 Snack
25 cashews and 1 grapefruit

Meal 4 Snack
20 almonds and 2 egg whites and 1 apple

Meal 5 Dinner
1 can tuna on English muffin and 1 cup greens

P.M. Snack (optional)
protein bar see appendix for best bars and snacks

The Body Type Diet: Combination Meals for Body Type 1, Bloated Fat

Water Balance	Water Balance	Water Balance	Water Balance
Breakfast	Lunch	Dinner	Snacks
▪ 1 cup cereal and 10 oz. milk and ½ cup berries (Kashi, Basic 4, Raisin Bran, Honey Nut Cheerios or Special K) ▪ 4 egg whites and ½ cucumber on a pita ▪ Spanish omelet (3 eggs, ½ cup veggies, 1 cheese and 3 tsp. salsa) ▪ 8 oz. ground turkey and ½ cup chili and ¼ cup brown rice ▪ 4 egg whites and 1 cup honeydew and watermelon	▪ 8 oz. chicken in wrap with 1 tomato ▪ hamburger in a salad with 1 apple ▪ 4 egg whites and 2 slices turkey and 1 cup pineapple ▪ 6 tsp. peanut butter on 2 slices whole grain and 6 oz. cottage cheese ▪ 1 cup oatmeal and 15 grapes and 2 egg whites	▪ 8 oz. chicken and 1 sliced apple and 1 pear in a salad ▪ 20 grapes in a salad with 5 egg whites ▪ 8 oz. lean steak and 1 sweet potato and 3 tbsp. sunflower seeds ▪ 1 can tuna in a salad with 1 cup pineapple ▪ 1 turkey burger and 1 cup spinach and 1 cup apple sauce	▪ 8 oz. cottage cheese and 15 grapes ▪ 1 cup watermelon and 1 string cheese ▪ 8 oz. yogurt and 20 grapes ▪ 2 graham crackers with 6 tsp. peanut butter ▪ 20 grapes and 2 slices cheese and 2 slices turkey

The Body Type Diet: Combination Meals for Body Type 1, Bloated Fat

Weight Loss	Weight Loss	Weight Loss	Weight Loss
Breakfast	Lunch	Dinner	Snacks
• 3 pieces dark choco-late and 20 grapes and 4 slices turkey • 8 oz. yo-gurt and 15 grapes and 20 almonds • 1 cup oat-meal and 1 cup berries • 4 egg whites and 1 cup greens • 2 whole grain waffles and 1 8 oz. yogurt • Melt or Shape pro-tein shake	• 1 can tuna and 20 pistachios and 4 tbsp. brown rice and 3 tsp. low-fat salad dressing • 4 slices turkey on English muf-fin with 1 red pepper • 4 slices roast beef and 1 grape-fruit and 15 almonds • 1 can tuna in a salad with 1 hard-boiled egg • 5 egg whites on whole grain (2 slices) with 1 tomato	• 2 egg whites and 4 fig newtons • 8 oz. yogurt and 1 cup grape nuts • 20 almonds and 20 yo-gurt-covered raisins • Protein shake (can) (25 grams of pro-tein) and 5 strawberries • 1 red pep-per and 2 slices low-fat cheese	• 8 oz. cottage cheese and 15 grapes and 4 tbsp. pine nuts • 1 cup water-melon and 2 string cheese and 2 egg whites • 8 oz. yo-gurt and 12 grapes and 10 cashews • 15 Wheat Thins and 6 tsp. cream cheese • Small bag of pretzels and 6 tsp. peanut butter

DAY-BY-DAY EATING PLAN FOR BODY TYPE 2, SOFT FAT
(WITH RECIPES)

MONDAY

Meal 1 Breakfast
Blend Lean or Athlete protein shake

Meal 2 Lunch
5 tsp. peanut butter and 8 oz. yogurt and 10 cashews

Meal 3 Snack
15 grapes and 2 slices turkey and 3 tbsp. sunflower seeds

Meal 4 Snack
1 cup raw veggies and 4 tsp. cream cheese

Meal 5 Dinner
8 oz. chicken and 1 baked potato and 1 cup greens

P.M. Snack (optional)
1 cup applesauce

DAY-BY-DAY EATING PLAN FOR BODY TYPE 2, SOFT FAT
(WITH RECIPES)

TUESDAY

Meal 1 Breakfast
Blend Lean or Athlete protein shake

Meal 2 Lunch
1 turkey burger and 1 cup applesauce

Meal 3 Snack
15 almonds and 7 yogurt pretzels

Meal 4 Snack
4 tsp. peanut butter and 2 celery sticks

Meal 5 Dinner
8 oz. fresh fish and 1 cup pineapple

P.M. Snack (optional)
1 rice cake and 2 egg whites

Day-By-Day Eating Plan for Body Type 2, Soft Fat
(with recipes)

Wednesday

Meal 1 Breakfast
Blend Lean or Athlete protein shake

Meal 2 Lunch
4 slices roast beef on 2 slices rye and 10 walnuts

Meal 3 Snack
3 tbsp. sunflower seeds and 8 oz. cottage cheese

Meal 4 Snack
1 apple and 15 Wheat Thins

Meal 5 Dinner
8 oz. ground beef and 3 egg whites and ¼ cup melted cheese

P.M. Snack (optional)
3 tsp. peanut butter and 3 tsp. jelly

DAY-BY-DAY EATING PLAN FOR BODY TYPE 2, SOFT FAT
(WITH RECIPES)

THURSDAY

Meal 1 Breakfast
Blend Lean or Athlete protein shake

Meal 2 Lunch
1 can tuna and 1 cup pineapple and 15 cashews

Meal 3 Snack
protein bar or snack see appendix

Meal 4 Snack
15 almonds and 1 peach

Meal 5 Dinner
8 oz. fresh fish and 1 baked potato and 1 cup spinach

P.M. Snack (optional)
10 grapes and 2 slices low-fat cheese

Day-By-Day Eating Plan for Body Type 2, Soft Fat
(with recipes)

Friday

Meal 1 Breakfast
Blend Lean or Athlete protein shake

Meal 2 Lunch
1 veggie burger and 1 cup brown rice

Meal 3 Snack
4 dried figs and 20 almonds and 10 grapes

Meal 4 Snack
1 cup raw vegetables and 5 tsp. peanut butter

Meal 5 Dinner
1 8 oz. lamb chop and 1 cup applesauce and 1 cup greens

P.M. Snack (optional)
2 rice cakes with 4 tsp. cream cheese

Day-By-Day Eating Plan for Body Type 2, Soft Fat
(with recipes)

Saturday

Meal 1 Breakfast
Protien yogurt or muffin or oatmeal see appendix

Meal 2 Lunch
1 8 oz. sirloin burger on 2 slices whole grain

Meal 3 Snack
2 fig newtons and 15 almonds and 1 apple

Meal 4 Snack
1 cup melon and 1/2 cup peanuts

Meal 5 Dinner
8 oz. chicken breast and 2 cups greens

P.M. Snack (optional)
1 graham cracker and 4 tsp. peanut butter

Day-By-Day Eating Plan for Body Type 2, Soft Fat

Sunday

Meal 1 Breakfast
1 cup melon or an orange and 20 cashews

Meal 2 Lunch
1 can tuna and 1 cup greens and 10 almonds

Meal 3 Snack
½ cup dried fruit and 2 slices turkey

Meal 4 Snack
1 red bell pepper and 15 almonds

Meal 5 Dinner
sushi or sashimi (6 rolls and 4 pieces sashimi)

P.M. Snack (optional)
apple and 10 almonds

The Body Type Diet: Combination Meals for Body Type 2, Soft Fat

Complete Athlete	Complete Athlete	Complete Athlete	Complete Athlete
Breakfast	Lunch	Dinner	Snacks
<ul><li>3 egg whites and 2 slices turkey and 2 tbsp. pine nuts</li><li>5 egg whites and ½ tomato and ½ potato</li><li>4 egg whites and 8 oz. chicken breast and ½ cup brown rice</li><li>4 egg whites and 2 slices cheese in a pita</li><li>5 egg whites and 3 oz. steak and ½ sweet potato</li><li>Lean Blend shake</li></ul>	<ul><li>3 slices turkey and 2 egg whites and 1 grapefruit</li><li>6 oz. steak and salad and apple</li><li>3 egg whites and 3 slices turkey in a pita</li><li>5 slices turkey in a salad with 3 tbsp. pine nuts</li><li>protein pita (see recipes)</li></ul>	<ul><li>3 fig newtons and 20 almonds</li><li>Zone bar or Balance gold bar</li><li>8 oz. cottage cheese and 20 cashews</li><li>15 Wheat Thins and 3 slices turkey</li><li>15 almonds and 15 cashews and 15 M&M's and ¼ cup dried fruit</li></ul>	<ul><li>apple and 3 slices turkey</li><li>tomato and 2 slices cheese</li><li>peach or plum and 20 almonds</li><li>pear and 3 tbsp. sunflower seeds</li><li>8 oz. yogurt and 8 oz. cottage cheese</li><li>Athlete or Lean Blend shake</li></ul>

The Body Type Diet: Combination Meals for Body Type 2, Soft Fat

Sports Performance	Sports Performance	Sports Performance	Sports Performance
Breakfast	Lunch	Dinner	Snacks
▪ 3 egg whites and 1 cup oatmeal ▪ breakfast quiche (see recipes) ▪ 4 egg whites and 2 slices turkey and 1 cup greens ▪ Protein shake – 50 grams (see recipes) ▪ Protein oatmeal (see recipes) ▪ Athlete or Lean Blend shake	▪ 3 slices turkey and 2 egg whites and 1 grapefruit ▪ 6 oz. steak and salad and apple ▪ 3 egg whites and 3 slices turkey in a pita ▪ 5 slices turkey in a salad with 3 tbsp. pine nuts ▪ protein pita (see recipes)	▪ protein French toast (see recipes) ▪ protein wraps (see recipes) ▪ 1 turkey burger and 1 sweet potato and 10 almonds ▪ hot roast beef plate (see recipes) ▪ power pancakes (see recipes)	▪ 20 cashews and 20 almonds ▪ 1 pear and 5 slices turkey ▪ 1 cup fruit salad and 25 pistachios ▪ 4 tbsp. sunflower seeds in 8 oz. yogurt ▪ 8 oz. yogurt and 1 cup berries and 15 cashews ▪ Athlete or Lean protein shake

Day-By-Day Eating Plan for Body Type 3, Solid Fat

Monday

Meal 1 Breakfast

Melt or Shape Blend shake

Meal 2 Lunch

4 slices roast beef and 2 slices cheese on 2 slices wshole grain

Meal 3 Snack

3 slices turkey and 1 pear

Meal 4 Snack

1 cup raw veggies and 4 tsp. peanut butter

Meal 5 Dinner

power salad see apendix for recipe

P.M. Snack (optional)

10 almonds and 10 cashews

Day-By-Day Eating Plan for Body Type 3, Solid Fat
(with recipes)

Tuesday

Meal 1 Breakfast
Shape Blend shake

Meal 2 Lunch
4 turkey slices and 1 cup greens and 20 cashews

Meal 3 Snack
1 vitamin water and 20 cashews

Meal 4 Snack
1 apple and 15 pretzels

Meal 5 Dinner
1 can tuna and 25 Goldfish crackers in a salad

P.M. Snack (optional)
protein bar see appendix

DAY-BY-DAY EATING PLAN FOR BODY TYPE 3, SOLID FAT
(WITH RECIPES)

WEDNESDAY

Meal 1 Breakfast
Shape Blend shake

Meal 2 Lunch
2 cups greens and 8 oz. chicken breast

Meal 3 Snack
1 cup applesauce and 20 almonds

Meal 4 Snack
20 cashews and 3 slices low-fat cheese

Meal 5 Dinner
sirloin burger with 1/2 avocado and 1 piece of cheese

P.M. Snack (optional)
1 cup granola and 8 oz. plain yogurt

Day-By-Day Eating Plan for Body Type 3, Solid Fat
(with recipes)

Thursday

Meal 1 Breakfast
Melt Blend shake

Meal 2 Lunch
4 slices turkey and 2 slices cheese in a salad

Meal 3 Snack
1 peach or plum and 3 egg whites

Meal 4 Snack
3 fig newtons and 8 oz. low-fat milk

Meal 5 Dinner
8 oz. flank steak and 1 cup fruit salad

P.M. Snack (optional)
1 cup peaches or pears

**DAY-BY-DAY EATING PLAN FOR BODY TYPE 3, SOLID FAT
(WITH RECIPES)**

FRIDAY

Meal 1 Breakfast
Shape Blend shake

Meal 2 Lunch
1 can tuna and 1 cup pineapple

Meal 3 Snack
20 yogurt-covered raisins and 15 almonds

Meal 4 Snack
8 oz. yogurt and 2 slices turkey

Meal 5 Dinner
string bean chicken cashew stir fry (see recipes)

P.M. Snack (optional)
protein bar or snack see appendix

DAY-BY-DAY EATING PLAN FOR BODY TYPE 3, SOLID FAT
(WITH RECIPES)

SATURDAY

Meal 1 Breakfast
1 cup grits or oatmeal and 4 egg whites

Meal 2 Lunch
4 slices turkey and 2 slices cheese and 1 cup greens

Meal 3 Snack
4 figs and 20 cashews

Meal 4 Snack
1 pear and 15 almonds and 2 tbsp. sunflower seeds

Meal 5 Dinner
8 oz. leg of lamb and 1 cup mashed potatoes and salad

P.M. Snack (optional)
12 pretzels and 3 tsp. cream cheese

Day-By-Day Eating Plan for Body Type 3, Solid Fat
(with recipes)

Sunday

Meal 1 Breakfast
4 egg whites and 1 tomato on 2 slices whole wheat

Meal 2 Lunch
1 can tuna on 2 slices rye with sliced pear

Meal 3 Snack
1 cucumber and 3 slices turkey

Meal 4 Snack
1 tomato and 20 almonds

Meal 5 Dinner
8 oz. steak in a salad with 1 cup greens

P.M. Snack (optional)
1 small box raisins and 20 cashews

The Body Type Diet: Combination Meals for Body Type 3, Solid Fat

Fat Burning	Fat Burning	Fat Burning	Fat Burning
Breakfast	Lunch	• • Dinner •	Snacks
• apple and 8 oz. yogurt • Zone bar • protein shake (can) (25 grams protein) and 20 almonds and 10 raisins • 1 peach and 3 slices turkey • 2 pieces dark chocolate and 5 strawberries • Melt or Shape Blend shake	• 1 can tuna and 5 tbsp. brown rice and 20 pistachios and 3 tsp. dressing • Sliced pear and 4 tsp. hummus in pita • Sliced apple and 5 tsp. peanut butter on whole wheat (2 slices) • 1 cup oatmeal and 20 almonds and 1 tbsp. peanut butter • 1 tomato and 8 oz. chicken in a salad	• 1 tbsp. whey protein powder and 8 oz. cottage cheese and 4 slices of turkey • 8 oz. salmon in spinach salad and 1 tomato and ½ cucumber with 4 tsp. low-fat dressing • 8 oz. fresh fish and 1 grapefruit • 8 oz. lean burger in lettuce wrap and melted cheese (2 slices) • 8 oz. chicken and 1 sliced pear in 2 hard-shell tacos with 4 tsp. salsa	• 4 asparagus and 1 cucumber • 12 oz. low-fat milk and 1 granola bar • 4 tbsp. sunflower seeds and 8 oz. cottage cheese • 12 pretzels and 6 tsp. peanut butter • Pear and 1 cup granola • Melt or Shape Blend shake

The Body Type Diet: Combination Meals for Body Type 3, Solid Fat

Thermogenic	Thermogenic	Thermogenic	Thermogenic
Breakfast	Lunch	Dinner	Snacks
<ul><li>1 tbsp. whey protein powder and 8 oz. cottage cheese</li><li>1 cup oatmeal and 20 almonds and 1 tbsp. peanut butter</li><li>20 grapes and 6 egg whites</li><li>2 English muffins with 6 tsp. peanut butter and 3 tsp. cream cheese</li><li>Fruit salad and 2 hard-boiled eggs</li><li>Shape Blend shake</li></ul>	<ul><li>Sliced pear and 4 tsp. hummus in pita</li><li>Sliced apple and 5 tsp. peanut butter on whole wheat (2)</li><li>1 cup oatmeal and 20 almonds and 1 tbsp. peanut butter</li><li>1 tomato and 8 oz. chicken in a salad</li><li>8 oz. chicken and 20 cashews and 1 cup greens (stir fry)</li></ul>	<ul><li>Green omelet (see recipes)</li><li>Pita and 1 can tuna and 3 rings pineapple</li><li>½ turkey sandwich (4 slices) and 2 apples</li><li>8 oz. flank steak and 1 kiwi in a salad</li><li>8 oz. chicken and 7 asparagus</li></ul>	<ul><li>4 asparagus and 1 cucumber</li><li>12 oz. low-fat milk and 1 granola bar</li><li>4 tbsp. sunflower seeds and 8 oz. cottage cheese and 1 piece dark chocolate</li><li>12 pretzels and 6 tsp. peanut butter and 15 grapes</li><li>1 red bell pepper and 15 cashews and 2 slices turkey</li><li>Melt Blend shake</li></ul>

Day-By-Day Eating Plan for Body Type 4, Skinny Fat

Monday

Meal 1 Breakfast
Nourish or Lean Blend shake

Meal 2 Lunch
8 oz. shredded chicken and 3 tsp. peanut butter on 2 slices whole grain

Meal 3 Snack
4 tsp. peanut butter and 20 cashews

Meal 4 Snack
12 almonds and protein brownie see appendix

Meal 5 Dinner
8 oz. sirloin burger and 1 cup brown rice with a salad

P.M. Snack (optional)
10 grapes and 2 slices cheese

DAY-BY-DAY EATING PLAN FOR BODY TYPE 4, SKINNY FAT
(WITH RECIPES)

TUESDAY

Meal 1 Breakfast
Nourish or Lean Blend shake

Meal 2 Lunch
create a salad (see appendix)

Meal 3 Snack
3 turkey slices and 1 grapefruit and 10 almonds

Meal 4 Snack
1 cup Honey Nut Cheerios and 8 oz. plain yogurt

Meal 5 Dinner
sushi or sashimi (6) rolls

P.M. Snack (optional)
2 1oz. pieces dark chocolate

Day-By-Day Eating Plan for Body Type 4, Skinny Fat

Wednesday

Meal 1 Breakfast
Nourish or Lean Blend shake

Meal 2 Lunch
Chinese steamed chicken and mixed vegetables

Meal 3 Snack
1 cup melon and 4 slices turkey

Meal 4 Snack
1 cup greens and 20 cashews

Meal 5 Dinner
8 oz. fresh fish and 1 grapefruit

P.M. Snack (optional)
1 apple or pear

DAY-BY-DAY EATING PLAN FOR BODY TYPE 4, SKINNY FAT
(WITH RECIPES)

THURSDAY

Meal 1 Breakfast
Nourish or Lean Blend shake

Meal 2 Lunch
2 English muffins with 6 tsp. peanut butter and jelly

Meal 3 Snack
3 fig newtons and 3 figs

Meal 4 Snack
½ cup dried fruit and 20 almonds

Meal 5 Dinner
1 turkey burger and 1 cup melon and 15 almonds

P.M. Snack (optional)
½ cup popcorn

DAY-BY-DAY EATING PLAN FOR BODY TYPE 4, SKINNY FAT
(WITH RECIPES)

FRIDAY

Meal 1 Breakfast
Nourish or Lean Blend shake

Meal 2 Lunch
1 can tuna and 3 tbsp. sunflower seeds and 1 apple

Meal 3 Snack
3 rice cakes with 6 tsp. jelly

Meal 4 Snack
2 carrot sticks and 20 cashews

Meal 5 Dinner
8 oz. chicken breast and 1 cup applesauce and 1 cup of greens

P.M. Snack (optional)
1 cup shredded wheat cereal and 8 oz. milk

Day-By-Day Eating Plan for Body Type 4, Skinny Fat
(with recipes)

Saturday

Meal 1 Breakfast
4 egg whites and 1 cup applesauce

Meal 2 Lunch
3 slices turkey and 3 slices roast beef and 2 slices low-fat cheese
in a salad

Meal 3 Snack
4 dried figs and 2 tbsp. sunflower seeds

Meal 4 Snack
3 pieces dark chocolate and 20 grapes

Meal 5 Dinner
protein pizza (see appendix)

P.M. Snack (optional)
10 pretzels

DAY-BY-DAY EATING PLAN FOR BODY TYPE 4, SKINNY FAT
(WITH RECIPES)

SUNDAY

Meal 1 Breakfast
grilled cheese delight (see appendix)

Meal 2 Lunch
big salad with choice of protein (8 oz. chicken or 5 egg whites)

Meal 3 Snack
20 pistachios and 8 oz. yogurt

Meal 4 Snack
1 red   bell pepper and 20 cashews

Meal 5 Dinner
8 oz. salmon in a salad with 1 cup pineapple

P.M. Snack (optional)
2 graham crackers

The Body Type Diet: Combination Meals for Body Type 4, Skinny Fat

Hormonal	Hormonal	Hormonal	Hormonal
Breakfast	Lunch	Dinner	Snacks
• 25-gram protein shake and 15 grapes • 3 egg whites and 1 orange • 1 grape-fruit and 20 cashews • apple and 20 raisins and 3 slices turkey • Balance gold bar and 10 almonds • Nourish or Lean Blend shake	• 8 oz. chicken in a salad with 3 tsp. dressing and 5 tbsp. sun-flower seeds • 8 oz. steak and 1 potato and 1 cup cauliflower • 8 oz. pastra-mi and 1 cup brown rice and 1 tomato • protein French fries (see recipes) • Lettuce wraps with 8 oz. turkey burger and 1 cup peaches	• 2 slices cheese and 1 tomato on 2 slices whole grain • 5 tsp. hum-mus and pear and 2 egg whites • Lean steak and 1 cup fruit salad in a salad with 3 tsp. dressing • 8 oz. chicken and 2 egg whites and 1 apple • 1 can tuna and 1 cup applesauce	• 8 oz. yogurt and 1 cup granola and ¼ cup hazelnuts • 3 slices tur-key and 1 apple and 10 almonds • Zone bar and 2 egg whites • 3 egg whites and 2 slices turkey • 2 slices tur-key and 2 slices roast beef and 1 tomato • Nourish or Lean Blend shake

The Body Type Diet: Combination Meals for Body Type 4, Skinny Fat

Tone N Tighten	Tone N Tighten	Tone N Tighten	Tone N Tighten
Breakfast	Lunch	Dinner	Snacks
<ul><li>1 cup hot cereal and 5 tsp. peanut butter and 1 hard-boiled egg</li><li>whole grain English muffin with 6 tsp. cream cheese and 1 apple</li><li>1 cup melon and 10 oz. cottage cheese</li><li>2 slices whole wheat and 6 tsp. peanut butter</li><li>1 cup oatmeal and 4 egg whites and 10 almonds</li><li>Lean or Tighten Blend shake</li></ul>	<ul><li>Lettuce wraps with 8 oz. turkey burger and 1 cup peaches</li><li>Pita with 4 slices cheese and 1 apple</li><li>8 oz. of 2% Fage yogurt and 20 pistachios and 1 tbsp. honey</li><li>8 oz. steak and 3 egg whites in a salad with 3 tsp. dressing</li><li>tuna melt (see recipe)</li></ul>	<ul><li>8 oz. chicken in a salad with 3 tsp. dressing and 5 tbsp. sunflower seeds</li><li>8 oz. steak and 1 potato and 1 cup cauliflower</li><li>8 oz. fresh fish and 1 tomato</li><li>(2) 6 oz. veggie burgers and 1 cup applesauce</li><li>7 tbsp. hummus in a pita with 1 sliced pear</li></ul>	<ul><li>1 vitamin water and 3 egg whites</li><li>8 oz. cottage cheese and 25 pistachios</li><li>3 slices turkey and 1 red bell pepper</li><li>1 cucumber and 1 tomato</li><li>1 kiwi and 4 slices turkey</li><li>Lean or Tighten Blend shake</li></ul>

The Body Type Diet: Combination Meals for All Body Types

Salt and Sugar (all body types) replace any meals	Basic Nutrient (all body types) replace any meals
orange and 2 slices low-fat cheese • 1 vitamin water and small bag of chips • 2 pieces of dark chocolate and ½ cup peanuts • ½ cup peanuts and 1 cup applesauce • small bag of baked potato chips and 1 orange • 10 pretzel sticks and 4 tsp. peanut butter • 1 cup berries and 2 salted rice cakes • 8 oz. cottage cheese and 8 oz. yogurt • peach or plum and 4 tbsp. sunflower seeds • 4 fig newtons and 15 salted almonds • 20 grapes and 3 slices turkey and 1 piece dark chocolate • 1 cup pineapple and small bag of cheese doodles • 4 chocolate chip cookies and 20 salted cashews • 1 0z.dark chocolate bar and 10 almonds • 1 corn muffin and glass of 12 oz. milk • any Blend protein shake	8 oz. chicken and ½ cup rice and 1 cup green beans 3 egg whites and 1 English muffin and 1 slice low-fat cheese 8 oz. steak and 1 potato and 1 cup broccoli 3-egg salad on rye (2 slices) 8 oz. chicken and 1 potato and 1 cup greens 2 waffles and 2 egg whites and 1 cup frozen yogurt salad with 3 egg whites, 3 slices turkey, 3 slices roast beef, 2 slices cheese 4 slices turkey and 2 slices cheese on whole wheat (2) 6 tsp. peanut butter and 6 tsp. jelly on whole wheat (2) grilled chicken wrap (8 oz. chicken) 1 can tuna salad on rye (2) 3 tsp. light mayo 1 red bell pepper with 8 oz. cottage cheese and 3 tbsp. sunflower seeds pepper steak combo (see recipes) egg-white combo (see recipes) 8 oz. fresh fish and 1 cup greens and 1 apple any Blend protein shake

Chapter 7

———⊂⊃———

Living the Body Type Lifestyle

Dining out and business travel

You are dining out and you are immediately served bread and butter. Say, "No thank you." What your body first ingests is what it primarily fuels. Translation, if I eat the carbohydrates from the bread, no matter what good protein I eat, my body is going to go back to the carbohydrates from the bread for its food-combining power. The protein is therefore wasted. The second thing served is usually the salad, which provides high fiber before dinner, which is backward! Salad helps you process food, so you want it at the end of the meal. Salad provides insoluble fiber and is meaningless unless you have plenty of water and active enzymes present in your system. Without this environment, it will just make you bloated when you eat your dinner. Go the European route and have your salad with dinner or after dinner.

What you ingest first is a high-quality protein, then green veggies, and then you can add some carbohydrate, such as rice, potatoes, or whole -grain bread, and *then* add a salad. By eating like this you are working with the science of your body and proper food combining. Recap: give your body a good source of protein, which equals high amino acid power. You then eat some clean diuretic green vegetables, which get rid of excess salt, sugar, and water. You then can enjoy some carbohydrates, which help shape and strengthen your muscles. THEN have a nice salad for the fiber that helps the body process the meal effectively. Always drink plenty of water with your meals and after. Trust me, you will feel better eating like this. If you want dessert or alcohol, it's not a problem. Just drop your carbohydrates at dinner and replace them with a dessert. Or you can double your protein portion by simply adding two tablespoons of sunflower seeds to your meal or ten almonds and still enjoy dessert.

Business Travel

There is no reason to eat much differently than normal when you are traveling. It is always a good idea to include sports performance meals such as bars or shakes, which will help keep you lean and get rid of excess salt and sugar.

What I do is bring a little cooler or Tupperware container of my food. If you cannot make you own food, it's a good idea to choose whole-grain sandwiches of turkey and cheese or tuna fish. What will tend to happen is you will be in such a routine of eating frequently that you might get upset if you miss meals, and that's fine. As long as you continuously give your best effort, that is all I can ask of you.

All I want you to remember is that each time you miss a meal you are losing lean tissue, and you will slowly gain weight. If you can remember this fact, you will never go wrong when you travel. It is always a good idea to pack my sports performance trail mix that consists of fifteen almonds, fifteen cashews, and 1 oz. dark chocolate, which will trigger a fat-burning effect in your body. Remember whole foods is your primary choice, but you can always have a meal replacement shake, which is where my custom Blends come in handy for you. I have single serving packets of my blends for travel. Now we have no excuses to miss meals or make poor choices when we travel.

When all else fails, please remember to try to get protein over carbohydrates. If there is a shake bar or juice bar, just get a healthy shake mixed with whey protein powder and berries or peanut butter.

SNACKS ON THE GO

Here are ten great snacks to pack on the go that can replace any of your snack meals:

1. raw veggies and 20 almonds
2. 15 almonds and 15 cashews and 3 tbsp. sunflower seeds
3. 3 rice cakes and small box of raisins
4. 1 grapefruit and 20 pistachios
5. 15 Wheat Thins and 2 string cheese
6. 8 oz. cottage cheese and 1 cup mixed fruit salad
7. small bag of pretzels and 1 apple
8. 1 cup applesauce and 2 pieces dark chocolate
9. sports bar such as power crunch, rx bar or one basix
10. protein bar or power muffin or protein cookie (list of best bars, etc., will be provided)

Helpful Tips

1. If you drink alcohol, you want to break down the sugar in the alcohol so it's not stored primarily as fat in your body. All you have to do is keep a higher amino acid profile in your blood. To do this, I offer my own amino acid mix called stacked. Take one scoop of it in water, either before or after you drink or twelve almonds or two tablespoons of sunflower seeds, and combine any of those with alcohol, and you have found the trick to burn it off more efficiently. I am not giving you the green light to drink freely. Instead I am

being realistic, as we need to be able to live and enjoy life and be healthy at the same time.

2. If you do eat fast food, now you will know a trick for how to rid your body of most of it. You can get about 85% of that meal to leave your body more readily by just ingesting one to one and a half liters of water within a one-half-hour time span after eating. During this time, you might be bloated and full, but because it takes the body about two to three hours to start breaking down any meal, the immediate intake of water will cause the bad nutrients to leave your body quickly before they hit your digestive system.

3. At times we have bad days and resort to eating poorly based on emotions, be it excitement or sadness or fear. Regardless, the food choices surely aren't going to be in accordance with your plan. Let's say you had a few consecutive bad meals and you are probably feeling like you let yourself down. Don't worry. Remember that you have built a strong nutritional base, which means your body has all the right nutrients and all the right amino acids present in your bloodstream, so any excess food or bad food choices will be more readily burned. You do, however, need to be aware that you will experience more dramatic weight fluctuations when you eat erratically, because you will have created a very clean blood state. As a result, your body will react very differently to bad foods and cause a major increase in your weight. But don't worry There is more good news. Be thankful that your body will react like this, because it will allow you to fix it quickly. All you have to do to get back to your weight is drink extra water, like two liters, and all that fluid will get rid of all that junk and your weight will go back to your baseline weight. This is precisely why you can keep losing weight and why you'll keep the weigh off.

4. Fish and carbohydrates do not mix well. A classic example of this poor combination is sushi. Although it is still effective, the reality is this: if you want to drop weight quickly, eat fish and green veggies alone with no carbohydrates, which will enable the potassium and omega 3s in the fish to do their job of tightening your body. Limit the amount of fish you eat with carbohydrates because carbohydrates inhibit the function of the potassium and omega 3 fats, and the nutrients are therefore more readily stored than burned.

Chapter 8

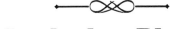

Body by Blend
Supplementation

I have developed my own supplement line called Blend and have also developed specific whey protein blends to incorporate into your meal plans for each specific body type.

I also have my first performance shake bar located at 213 Brook Street, Scarsdale, New York 10583.

I highly recommend customized monthly supplement kits for each body type, because they further assist you on your weight-loss journey.

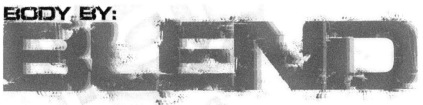

What is Body by Blend?

Body by Blend is a complete performance shake bar—be healthy, get fit, perform better. Incorporated in Body by Blend is a complete all-natural supplement line and complete nutritional program called The Body Type Diet. Although Blend is a nutrition-al supplement line, Blend also encompasses what I call complete wellness, because your body needs proper *nutrition* and *supple-mentation*, proper *exercise* and *motivation*.

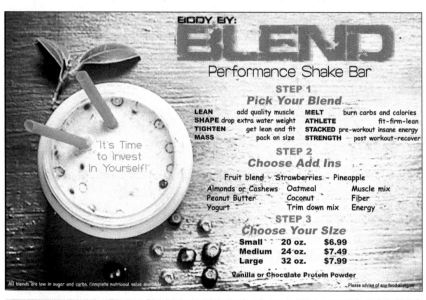

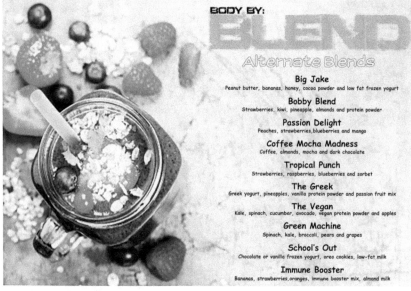

Having worked as a nutritionist, personal trainer, and motivational speaker over the years, I learned that people need to have two things to get fit. Number one, they need the will, and number two, they need the right way, which is where Blend steps in to show you the right way for your individual body type. You must have the right tools and knowledge. When I take on clients, I help them by putting them on a program, ranging from two to six months, depending on what I think they need.

The best investment you will ever make in your life is to decide to invest in yourself! "Destiny is not a matter of chance but rather a matter of choice."

The fact that you are reading this book now shows your commitment and integrity. Consider me your Body by Blend coach. I will be with you every step of the way.

Body by Blend is located at 213 Brook Street, Scarsdale, New York 10583
email blend183@yahoo.com
instagram blend183
723-9100

ROBERT ADAMO

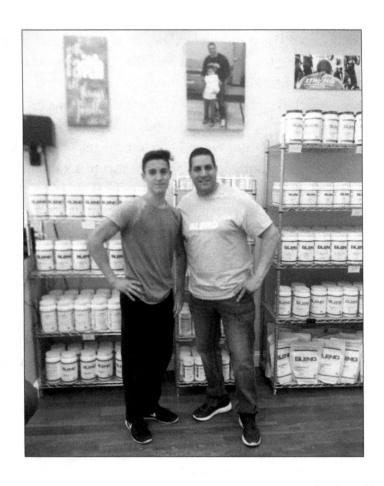

Acknowledgments

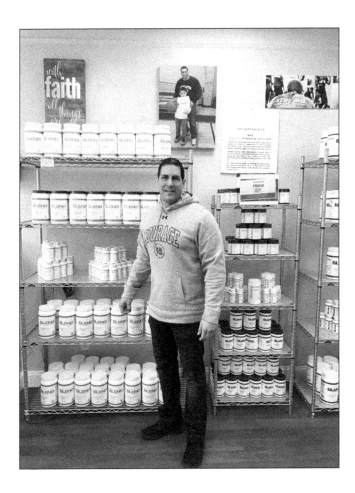

Many people over the years have enabled this project to come true finally. My dad once told me, "When you put God first in your life, you will never finish second." During the times when I struggled, times when it was tough for me to persevere, I gave my faith and found my strength in the Good Lord.

I want to thank the Good Lord above for enabling many dreams of mine to come true.

To everyone who helped me along the way, financially and emotionally, I want to say thanks.

Mel Berger, thank you for all your positive feedback over the years and telling me, "I think we have a book here."

My three sons, Robbie, Rocco, and Jake, I love you dearly.

My three beautiful sisters Ann, Laura, and Amy, love you lots. Laura, for all our talks and you making sure I followed the Lord and stayed on my path, I love you for that. Amy, for the times when you were there for me when I needed help, I love you.

Mom and Dad, it hasn't been easy raising me, but I've appreciated all your love.

Richard Perez Feria, you were an amazing inspiration to me.

Andy Behrman, you helped me so much in my journey with this book. Thank you!

Kelly Jones, who made my supplement line Blend come true, big thanks.

All the Eastchester Sanitation crew, Jeff "Denzel," thanks for all the talks—my therapist at times. You're the best. Big Ant, Damon, love you for all the laughs, especially Chili man Mark Garofola, always shaking me down for chili money!

The Eastchester police, Steve "The LEG" Dilege, and Nick "the hammer" Louros, thanks for your great support.

Adamo, with a name like that you are the best! Thanks for being a great friend along with my man Chas, Burrata rocks.

The Eastchester Fire Department, especially Kenny Simonides, you came through for me at a time I needed you most. Thanks for all your support. Eastchester EMS, big thanks.

Maria and Brian and Eastchester Town Hall, thanks for welcoming me!

Paresh and ABS Café Grill, thanks for making the best muffins ever.

Pizza man Otto and Hugo, big thanks. Even though you called me a muffin top, I'm still grateful.

Karen and Bobby Carinci, thank you for believing in me and supporting Blend.

Carlo, my Gumba and best hair stylist, thank you for looking out for me and sending me new customers. You're the best!

All my clients over the years who have touched my life completely, so proud of you!

Rob Corbi from Paychex, thanks for all your help and some great laughs.

Max from UPS, thank you for giving me the slogan, "Changing the Game."

Chris Jackson, we hit it off from day one. Thanks for all your support and belief in Blend.

I could probably go on forever and say thanks to so many people.

I put all my faith in God, and he recently sent me an angel, someone who loves me, accepts me, and totally understands me. The day I met you, Barbara, you took my breath away. Never has someone loved me so unconditionally. Barbara, they say that behind every great man is a great woman. You're that woman. I will forever remember and appreciate your beauty, kindness, and unbelievable faith and support in me. The days when you fought for us, even when I battled you, makes what we have so special. Telling you I love you more and more every day isn't quite enough. We are very blessed. My angel, super preemie, moo shoo, frazy nut, and pikachu. Your brother Vinny's life was taken away at a young age, but I know every time I find pennies and feathers, it's Vinny who is smiling down from Heaven and is so happy for you!

Finally, to all you readers who waited patiently for this book. You know it's been my lifelong commitment and mission to help others live a better, happier, and healthier life.

There are many more books to follow, and I hope all you folks stay with me and allow me to motivate and help you. I am grateful, grateful every day for the wonderful life God has given me. God bless each one of you.

And to my new readers and new friends, thanks for joining me on this journey. Please share my vision and see your dream!

Appendix

Body Type Diet Authorized Food Chart

Proteins	Fats
▪ Chicken breast ▪ Sliced turkey, fresh turkey, ground turkey, turkey burger ▪ Flank steak, lean cut steak ▪ Tuna ▪ Fresh fish—haddock, flounder, halibut, swordfish, lobster, crab, salmon ▪ Protein powder (whey) ▪ Egg whites ▪ Lean ham ▪ Lean roast beef	Cashews, almonds, sunflower seeds, pine nuts Flax seed oil, sunflower oil, safflower oil Avocado Peanut butter Whole eggs Pistachios Cream cheese

Complex Carbs (starchy)	Complex carbs (fibrous)
• Whole grain, whole wheat bread • Whole wheat bagels • Pasta • Sweet potatoes/yams • Baked potatoes • Brown rice • Oatmeal • Cream of Wheat • Cream of Rice • Pita • Beans—red, kidney, pinto, lima • Red potatoes • Corn • Lentils • Chick peas • Hard-shell tacos • Couscous • Rice cakes	• Asparagus • Broccoli • Cauliflower • Lettuce • Cucumber • Tomato • Peppers • String beans • Green beans • Psyllium fiber • Artichokes • Spinach • Lettuce • Mushrooms • Eggplant • Celery • Zucchini • Brussel sprouts • Popcorn • High fiber cereal

Fruit	Dairy
• Grapefruit	• Fage greek yogurt (0% fat)
• Apple	• Dannon Light and Fit yogurt
• Pear	• Cottage cheese
• Melon (cantaloupe, honeydew, watermelon)	• Cheese (Alpine Lace)
• Strawberries, raspberries, blueberries	• String cheese
• Pineapple	• Laughing Cow cheese
• Kiwi	• Low fat cheese
• Grapes	• 1% or 2% milk
• Cherries	
• Oranges	
• Peaches	
• Plums	
• Nectarines	

RECIPES

Power Omelette
- 4 egg whites, 2 slices cheese, ½ avocado and 1 tomato

Green Omelette
- 3 eggs, spinach, broccoli and asparagus and 2 slices cheese

Egg white combo
- 5 egg whites, 1 tomato and 1 avocado

Protein yogurt
- 10 oz. Greek yogurt, 1 tablespoon honey and 12 pistachios or almonds

Protein pizza
- 2 whole grain English muffins, tomato sauce, mozzarella cheese and chicken

Tuna melt
- I can tuna, 1 tomato and melted cheese

Create a salad
- No lettuce, tomato, cucumber, avocado, sunflower seeds and fish or chicken

String bean cashew stir fry
- 1 cup string beans, ¼ cup cashews, chicken and any low sodium soy sauce

Protein French toast
- 2 slices any bread, mix 2 tablespoons melt protein powder with 4 eggs

Protein wrap
- Whole grain wrap with 4 slices turkey, sliced apple, 2 pieces cheese and ½ avocado

Protein oatmeal
- 1 cup steel cut oatmeal, 1/ cup blueberries, 2 tablespoons melt protein powder and 1 tablespoon and 1 tablespoon of low sugar preserves

Cobb salad
- Fish or chicken, avocado, apple or pear, almonds and tomato

Power pancakes
- Panic pancake mix with 2 tablespoons melt protein powder and turkey bacon optional

Protein pita
- 1 can tuna or 4 egg whites, 2 slices cheese and sliced apple and sliced almonds

Protein lettuce wrap
- Ground turkey, peppers, onions and sauce in 2 big pieces lettuce

Grilled cheese delight
- 2 slices whole grain 4 slices cheese and tomatoes

Pepper steak combo
- Skirt steak, peppers onions and avocado and 12 cashews

Protein muffin
- Available at Body by Blend in Scarsdale, New York

Breakfast quiche
- Almond flour, 4 eggs, cheese, onion, cayenne pepper and spinach

BARS and SNACKS

- Zing protein bars
- Combat protein bars
- Power crunch protein bars
- Zone bars
- BHU fit bars
- Owyn bars
- Kind bars
- Eat me guilt free brownies
- Enlightened bada beans
- Quest protein chips
- Good health sweet potato or apple chips
- Skinny dipped almonds

CPSIA information can be obtained
at www.ICGtesting.com
Printed in the USA
FFHW011721250219
50705127-56089FF